YOUR KNOWLEDGE HAS VALUE

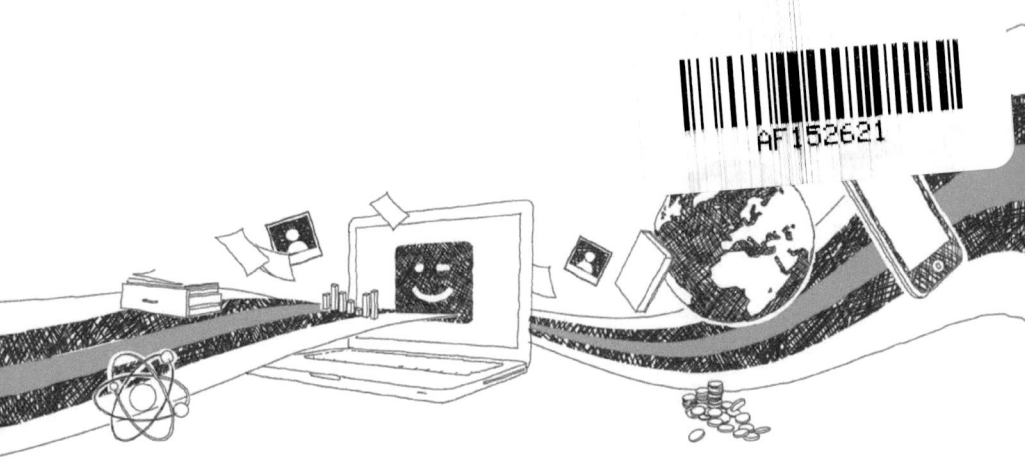
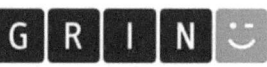

Marissa Tremblett

Searching Techniques in Forensic Anthropology

GRIN Verlag

Bibliografische Information der Deutschen Nationalbibliothek:

Die Deutsche Bibliothek verzeichnet diese Publikation in der Deutschen National-
bibliografie; detaillierte bibliografische Daten sind im Internet über http://dnb.d-
nb.de/ abrufbar.

Dieses Werk sowie alle darin enthaltenen einzelnen Beiträge und Abbildungen
sind urheberrechtlich geschützt. Jede Verwertung, die nicht ausdrücklich vom
Urheberrechtsschutz zugelassen ist, bedarf der vorherigen Zustimmung des Verla-
ges. Das gilt insbesondere für Vervielfältigungen, Bearbeitungen, Übersetzungen,
Mikroverfilmungen, Auswertungen durch Datenbanken und für die Einspeicherung
und Verarbeitung in elektronische Systeme. Alle Rechte, auch die des auszugsweisen
Nachdrucks, der fotomechanischen Wiedergabe (einschließlich Mikrokopie) sowie
der Auswertung durch Datenbanken oder ähnliche Einrichtungen, vorbehalten.

Imprint:

Copyright © 2014 GRIN Verlag GmbH
Druck und Bindung: Books on Demand GmbH, Norderstedt Germany
ISBN: 978-3-656-68662-0

This book at GRIN:

http://www.grin.com/en/e-book/275643/searching-techniques-in-forensic-anthropo-
logy

GRIN - Your knowledge has value

Der GRIN Verlag publiziert seit 1998 wissenschaftliche Arbeiten von Studenten, Hochschullehrern und anderen Akademikern als eBook und gedrucktes Buch. Die Verlagswebsite www.grin.com ist die ideale Plattform zur Veröffentlichung von Hausarbeiten, Abschlussarbeiten, wissenschaftlichen Aufsätzen, Dissertationen und Fachbüchern.

Visit us on the internet:

http://www.grin.com/

http://www.facebook.com/grincom

http://www.twitter.com/grin_com

REVIEW PAPER: SEARCHING TECHNIQUES IN FORENSIC ANTHROPOLOGY

FRSC 3900: Reading Course

Abstract

This report reviews the literature on the techniques used to locate human remains and clandestine graves that are used by forensic anthropologists and investigators. This paper critically examines multiple techniques including Human Remains Detection Dogs, Ground Penetrating Radar, Resistivity Surveys, Remote Sensing, Probing, Taphonomy, Soil Gas Survey and Civilian searches, to determine their advantages, disadvantages, reliability and credibility in locating clandestine graves. There is currently no one method that is successful in every condition and geographical location. But with the development of technology and with a multidisciplinary approach, researchers will be able to develop a method that will work in every condition in all geographical locations, help bettering law enforcement.

Marissa Tremblett

Inhalt

Introduction

This review covers a wide variety of forensic anthropological search techniques for human remains and clandestine graves. Clandestine graves are graves that are dug by an unknown person in an unknown location. It is one of the roles of forensic investigators and forensic anthropologists to help identify and locate human remains and these clandestine graves because without the victim's remains there would be a great deal of unsolved cases. Some suspects may not even see trial because there is no body for police agencies to link them to the crime. There are many techniques that can be used to locate these graves, ranging from older techniques, such as using human remains detection dogs, to newer techniques, such as using decompositional odor analysis. This review aims to look at a wide variety of different forensic anthropological searching techniques and identify how successful each of the techniques are for locating human remains and clandestine graves, and the limitations and problems of each technique. This review is based on the examination of the work of thirty-two articles and books that will cover all the areas of a number of different techniques currently being used in the field. A great majority of the articles are from academic peer reviewed journals, and range from the years 1995 to 2014.

Canines

Human remains detection dogs is one of the oldest (1) and reliable techniques for locating human remains and clandestine graves. A dogs' sense of smell is 1,000 times more sensitive than that of a human (2), which makes human remain detection (HRD) dogs a valuable asset when locating human remains and clandestine graves. But HRD dogs are not always accurate when it comes to locating human remains because they can often give "false alerts." Although HRD dogs can give false alerts, there are different external factors that can affect a HRD dog's ability to locating human remains, such as the amount and kind of training the dog has received, weather conditions, the strength of the scent, which might be lowered because there has been a long time since the victim's death, and other geological and ecological conditions (2). These factors are why HRD dogs undergo extensive training and continue to be tested regularly.

Training of HRD canines is curial to their ability and success out in the field. Lasseter et al.'s study of Cadaver dog and handler team capabilities in the recovery of buried human remains in the southeastern United States concluded that there needs to be standardization of how human remain detection dogs are trained (3). Not having a set of universal standards to train HRD dogs, hinders the HRD dog's credibility and reliability of locating human remains. Over the last decade there has been a push for set standardized techniques for training human remain detections dogs. Committees such as the Scientific Working Group for Dogs and Orthogonal Detector Guidelines (SWGDOG) have established what they believe to be the best practice guidelines for HRD dogs (1). SWGDOG consists of experts from local, state, federal and international agencies, who meet to determine these guidelines and explore how this discipline could be improved upon (1).

Along with this push, there have been recent developments to help and test the dog's accuracy; such developments include using volatile organic compounds (VOCs) to develop tools such as the Scent Transfer Unit (STU-100) (1) to help dogs get a better, stronger scent. VOCs are volatile organic compounds that come from the ground and the area surrounding human remains in a grave (4). They are incredibly useful for helping human remains detection dogs because they can make up whole odor profiles for the dogs to use. What is meant by this is that, when a body is decomposing it undergoes four known stages, Fresh (autolysis), Bloat (putrefaction), Decay (putrefaction and scavenging) and finally Dry (diagenesis or mummification) (5). Recently discovered, it will also release different scents, VOCs, at these stages. By understanding what VOCs are and the ability to provide the scent to the HRD dogs through technologies like the STU-100, dogs will now have a better capability of detecting the scent of human remains no matter what stage of decomposition they are in.

The Scent Transfer Unit is a "dynamic airflow collection device" (1). The STU-100 takes the scent from the sample you want the dog to get the scent from and concentrates it, so they can get a stronger, amplified scent to work from (1). The whole system is made up of a Teflon-coated hood, which holds a gauze pad that collects the concentrated scent from the sample that is attached to a small vacuum pump. The air from the vacuum draws the scent from the sample, to the gauze pad which holds the concentrated VOC, which then can be given to the dog to smell. This device has appeared to be very successful, showing that it has had success rates of 73.5% to 82.2% (1) from studies of it used in the field.

There have been similar studies that have explored the use of VOCs to advance the field in cadaver dogs. There has been research in Decompositional Odor Analysis (DOA) to help canines locate human remains. Currently there has been research done to make a database of

Decompositional Odor Analysis Volatile Organic Components. Creating this database has shown, researchers that the odors that come from decomposition changes over time (4). To be able to detect these changes of scents, the researchers have developed different methods and techniques to collect these samples. Such methods include Triple Sorbent Traps and the Spiking method.

The Triple Sorbent Traps (TSTs) are made up of sections of 14mm Carbotrap-C, Carbosieve S-III sorbents that are packed into a stainless steel tube (4). Once the sorbents are placed in the tube, the Triple Sorbent Traps are cleaned by being heated to 380°C for approximately three to four hours long (4). During this process there is a flow of helium that is introduced at 50-100mL/min to further clean them. After the traps are cleaned they are stored in a freezer at -18°C (4). These traps are used by being put into the ground, via the spiking method. The Spiking Method consists of a static dilution process that utilizes 250 mL amber dilution bottles; which are equipped with a screw-on vapor-lock valved cap; which is constantly maintained between 70°C to 90°C during this process (4). The Spiking method and the TSTs are used together to collect the VOCs from the sample area. These methods have produced great results by identifying 30 key makers of human decomposition (4). The discovery of these 30 makers proves to be important because they do not only add to the database of VOCs, but they are all detectable at the surface level of the grave, which makes it ideal for human remain detection dogs. This database is idea for human remains detection dogs because it allows for them to be better trained for remains at whatever decompositional stage.

Not only is technology helping HRD dogs to improve, in action experience is as well. HRD dog trainers and police forces are testing the dog's abilities in different circumstances by providing different types of training, such as in wildfire recoveries and searching for just human teeth. It is important to test HRD dogs in different circumstances because if there is problem where the dogs are not responding well because they the circumstance is preventing them to do so, the handlers can then train the HRD dogs to be able to respond to that circumstance. It is important to test the HRD dogs for searching areas of the body such as human teeth, because it shows that HRD are reliable for detecting human remains, even when they are locating the smallest of body parts.

Human teeth, are the strongest substance in the human body, they will often withstand extreme heat which makes them incredibly useful for identifying burnt human remains. But human teeth are small and often can be lost when the body is buried, moved or dumped. Training HRD dogs to locate all of the remains will prove advantageous, not only for credibility in the field but for identification purposes. Locating human teeth is not a standard in training HRD dogs and if a dog is to specifically locate human teeth the handler must train their dog to do so (6); this is the difficulty of not having this specific method standardized. The importance of finding teeth for identification purposes is important, and by not having the training could lead to not being able to identify an individual. Although this ability is valuable it is not well tested. There have been very little studies conducted on testing HRD on their ability to locate human teeth. One study done by Cablk et al. tested HRD abilities to locate teeth, but had a very small sample size, only having tested three dogs (6), that had different level of training. With having a small sample size it is hard to test the abilities objectively. Based on this study the dogs scored an 81%, 67% and 65% (6). The study does show that the HRD dogs can locate human teeth, and that with more testing we could get a better understanding of how reliable they can be for locating them.

Locating human teeth could prove very valuable especially in wildfire search and recoveries. Wildfires are naturally occurring fires that tend to be extremely large and have proven to be difficult to manage. They often burn down entire forests, and towns. It is unfortunate that sometime people who are living in these town, happen to be caught in the path of a wildfire, do not get the chance to evacuate and sometime die in these fires which is why HRD dogs are used in wildfire searches. Texas is an area that is prone to wildfires, and because of this they have created a task force, known as the Texas Task Force 1 Urban Search and Rescue (TX-TF1). The TX-TF1 uses HRD dogs to locate victims who were trapped in the way of the wildfire. In September of 2011, Texas was hit with an unsuspected wildfire that rapidly spread throughout Bastrop County. During and after this wildfire the TX-TF1 used HRD dogs in what is believed to be the largest detailed search for human remains (7) searching a final area of 15 598 acres (7) for human remains.

This research provides evidence of the importance and the abilities of HRD dogs in locating human remains. Dogs are one of the best of methods used for locating human remains; they are reliable and prove to have a great deal of success doing it even without the standardization. It is clear from the literature that canines are extremely successful at searching and locating human remains and clandestine graves, with standardization and more testing in areas such as locating human teeth, this technique of searching will only improve.

Geophysical

There are many different ways that technologies have been able to help forensic investigators locate human remains and clandestine graves. These techniques have proven to be extremely useful and successful at locating clandestine graves in different environments. Some of the most successful techniques the literature has indicated are Ground Penetrating Radar, Electrical Resistivity, Time-Lapse Resistivity, Remote Sensing and Probing.

Ground Penetrating Radar (GPR)

Ground Penetrating Radar (GPR) is without doubt the easiest and most used technological based searching technique that used to locate human remains and clandestine graves. GPR is commonly used in archaeological and forensic investigations because the units are portable, accurate, non-invasive, and non-destructive (8, 9). It has been a well-accepted method not only in the archaeology world but for forensic purposes since it was first successfully used in 1986 (9). GPR works by transmitting and reflecting Electromagnetic (EM) wave energy (2). A GPR survey is conducted with two antennas, the first one transmits the EM waves via short pulses into the ground while the other antenna receives the reflected waves (8) which provide a picture of what is going on underneath the surface when viewed on the display panel.

What makes GPR one of the more popular methods to use to locate clandestine graves is that the investigator collects data, from the survey, in real time, which can be displayed on a black & white or coloured screen (10). The investigators immediately know if they have found a possible location of a grave when looking at the real time data. Not only is GPR good for real time data, but it has the best resolution of subsurface features out of all the other geophysical technologies (10, 11). This advantage adds to why GPR is so popular to use to locate clandestine graves. From this real time data and the high resolution, investigators can make preliminary assessments from the field (10), and can start excavations immediately. The size and the depth of the grave can also be measured from the real time data (10) which allows the investigators to have an idea of what they are excavating, and to make sure they do not miss evidence. Finally what makes GPR so useful is that is can be used over concrete, blacktop and fresh water (10). This is advantageous because other methods may or cannot locate graves in these specific areas, but GPR can do this without disrupting the surface.

The majority of the literature on GPR support all these advantages and GPR also works well in conducive environments. There has been a lot of testing the use of GPR in other less friendly environments to see if it is just as accurate and reliable. The literature indicated that there are two main areas where GPR is not well tested, mountainous and coastal beach areas (9, 12).

Novo et al.'s study was a study that was used to test GPR in mountainous environments. The research team help Spanish Law Enforcement locate clandestine graves in mountainous environments using this method. To test the ability of 3D GPR Novo et al. research team buried two metal stakes one meter deep into the "grave" in a mountain environment. One stake was buried perpendicular to the surface and the other was buried orthogonally to the surface (9). The 3D GPR was conducted with a 250 MHz antenna (9), because it was a more robust, and would be able to with stand the mountainous environment without being damaged or broken. Along with the 250 MHz antenna they used GprMax software™ v.2.0 to create synthetic radar-grams which were used to test the ability of the antenna to detect the metal stakes (9). The research team ran into some problems that made it difficult to use the 3D-GPR, such as since they were in a mountainous environment they had to deal with performing the survey on very steep slopes. Along with the steep slope the team had to deal with the rugged terrain which made it difficult to make grids and conduct the survey (9). Although there were setbacks Novo et al. research team where able to get promising results back from their tests. They were able to complete their goal of finding both of the metal stakes, but the GPR was unsuccessful in distinguishing similar anomalies with the metal stakes (9). On top of this they were able, with careful analysis and review of the radar graphs, to use the graphs to exclude areas where the "grave" was less likely to be, showing that even unfavourable environments, such mountainous areas, GPR is still effective and reliable with locating clandestine graves.

There was another study that tested a different environment to see if GPR would still be effective at locating clandestine graves. There is approximately 440,000 km of coastline around the world and almost half of the world's population live within 100km of the coastline (12). Testing coastal beach environments is important since there is such a huge population that live in the vicinity of this environment. A beach environment might be ideal to spot to bury a body for a number of different reasons, one being is that loose sand is easier to dig than compact soil that have tree roots in it, like forest environments. Pringle et al. research team tested the ability of GPR and other geophysical technologies in this environment (12). They selected beaches based on whether they had direct beach access, close distance from main road, and areas that were not close to build-up or urban areas (12). These areas were selected because a suspect is more likely to bury a body in areas that are secluded and they have easy access to. To test the geophysical technologies the research team, buried fiber glass mannequins in three areas, the sandy area close to the water's edge, the grassy-sandy dune system, and the last one in between the two areas (12). All the graves were easily dug because the sand was saturated with enough water to prevent the grave walls from collapsing. After the graves where dug and reburied they searched the area with different geophysical techniques. They use GPR on three different frequencies, 225 MHz, 450 MHz and 900 MHz (12) to try and locate the "victims". Their researched distinguished that all three of the frequencies were successful in locating the mannequins, but noted that the 225 MHz was the most useful for searching this environments because it did not pick up as many non-target anomalies (12). They also noted that all the frequencies gave poor resolution, but frequency 450 MHz gave the best resolution out of the three (12). Finally Pringle et al.'s study concluded that the best frequency antenna for locating clandestine graves in costal beach environments was the 450MHz, but all three frequencies were successful able to locate the graves.

Studies like these suggest that GPR can be used to locate clandestine graves no matter the environment. There are current studies being done to test the ability of GPR to work in snow. The research team used an upwards-looking GPR to test the depth of the snow from when an avalanche occurs (13). Their study concluded that using 800-900MHz antennas, that GPR could successful test the depth of the snow cover (13). This study, could be applied to forensic investigations, although further testing would need to be done to test if the GPR could successful detect a grave through both the snow and ground.

These studies show that there is sufficient reliability when using GPR. Although GPR is reliable and very successful in locating clandestine grave, the technique is not perfect. There are a few disadvantages to using GPR such as the equipment is expensive to get, and it requires a specially trained technician to be able to use and interpret the images (10) reproduced by GPR. The skill of the operator is curial to the successfulness of the technique. The operator may mistake anomalies for a grave which will slow down the investigation because they will have to excavate it to confirm or reject the area. They also may consider evidence, like a gun, bullet casing and cell phones as anomalies and therefore they will never be collected (14). But with any technique human error is always a factor and the consistence testing will only make the technique better, accurate, and more reliable. Such testing like the original test done by Vaughan in 1986, is important because it test the accuracy and the reliability of GPR. Similar test have been conducted to test these key functions (8, 9) to ensure consistency.

Resistivity Surveys

Resistivity Surveys is an alternative method to GPR and HRD dogs for locating clandestine graves. It is best used when there has been a recent disturbance of the subsurface (2), but have also been effective in locating older graves. Resistivity Surveys have been tested to locate older graves in places like grave-yards where they have known graves (15) which ensure the credibility of the technique. It has also been proven to be very helpful in not only in forensic investigations but for locating unmarked burials in grave yards and ancient tombs (11). The electrical resistivity method locates clandestine graves by detecting the disturbance caused by initially excavating the grave and filling it back in. This disturbed soil is more porous, and therefore holds more water. The more water the soil holds changes the resistivity of the ground (16) which then can be detected by a resistivity survey. This technique is useful for locating clandestine graves, because when the body decomposes, the fluids go into the porous soil and increases the groundwater conductivity, which makes the grave detectable by the electrical resistivity survey (15, 16).

What makes Resistivity surveys a great technique for locating clandestine graves is that it can still detect the grave even if the victims is clothed, naked, or wrapped in a garbage bag or tarpaulin (15, 16). It is important to test to see is Resistivity Survey will still locate graves when the victim is wrapped in something whether it be clothes or a garbage bag because these materials can prevent or change how much decompositional fluid will diffuse in the surrounding soil (16). Knowing this is significant because Resistivity Surveys rely on the amount of fluid the soil is holding in order to get an exact reading (16). The literature shows that there have been studies on whether Resistivity Surveys can locate clandestine grave when they are wrapped.

To do a Resistivity Survey, you need to have a resistivity meter. One of the common meters used is called the Geoscan™ RM-15 (15). The Geoscan™ RM-15 is a multiplex resistivity meter that measures constant spaces of 0.5m. It has two probes what are spaced one meters apart, as well as a reference probe which are typically placed 16m away from the closest grid corner (15). In order to effectively use the resistivity meter the investigators need to set up a grid in the search area, this is important because the resistivity meter utilizes the grid line locating to make accurate scans of the area. Often other technologies such as Leica™ 1200 Real-Time Kinematic (RTK) differential Global Positioning Systems (dGPS) will be used to mark out grids, so that there are precise measurements (15). In addition to this investigators might have to mathematically calculate corner points of some of the grids to compensate for none movable objects for instance trees and large rocks (13). Finally technologies such as Generic Mapping Tools (GMT) software's can be used to assist the interpretation of the data, visually (16) so that investigator can get precise and accurate readings.

The advantage of using a resistivity meter is that is does not need a large team to complete the survey; huge areas can be surveyed by teams of two or more. Teams of two can cover huge areas for example 30m by 30m grids in three days, collecting as much as 21,667 sample points as indicated in one of the studies done (15). As well the Resistivity Survey appears to work even when other conventional methods such as HRD dogs and GPR have failed to locate anything (15).

Studies of the ability of Resistivity Surveys to locate clandestine graves when the victim is wrapped in materials have proven to be successful. These studied used pigs, as their "victims' because pigs are similar to humans in such as they have similar bones and decompose in similar ways (15). These pigs were wrapped in materials such as garbage bags and clothes, when the pigs where surveyed for, they were successfully found, no matter what they were wrapped in. The Resistivity Survey, based on the studies conducted, had proven successful in indicating all the pigs, but also showed other large anomalies that were close in size and depth (15, 16).

Other studies have been conducted that have tested Resistivity Survey abilities to located wrapped pigs over a three year period, to test its accuracy over time. This study looked at three different simulated clandestine graves, one pig was naked, the other pig was wrap in tarpaulin, and the last was an empty grave (17), to test if resistivity surveys could detect clandestine graves accurately after a three year period. Based on this study, the research team was able to successful, locate all three graves using resistivity surveys at all the various intervals throughout the three years. The study did conclude that the success of resistivity surveys detecting old clandestine graves was depended on the burial style the graves were dug (17). The study showed that out of the three graves, that the naked pig grave had a better chance of being discovered up to three years after the initial burial (17) than the wrapped pig. This was due to the amount of "fluids" that was leeched into the surrounding soil. Although the naked pig grave had a better chance of being discovered temporally, it did not mean that the wrapped pig could not be found three years after the initial burial. The study simply concluded that it would be more difficult, but not impossible, to locate the wrapped pig burial, because the wrapping prevented the fluid from leeching into the soil (17). The tightness of the wrapping of the pig plays a key role in the ability to locate the grave using resistivity surveys (17). The looser the wrapping is, the more fluid can escape and leech into the soil. When more fluid leeches into the soil, the better reading the resistivity survey because the survey work based of the amount of liquid that is in the ground.

Further research should be done to gain a better understanding of how the tightness of the wrapping, whether it be clothes, garbage bag or tarpaulin around a victim effects the amount of fluid that leeches into the soil. Once this factor is understood, it can be tested to make a better and more accurate resistivity survey that will better located wrapped victims in clandestine graves.

Remote Sensing

Remote Sensing is an alternative method for searching for clandestine graves. Using remote sensing as a method to locate clandestine graves will include methods such as aerial photography, topography mapping, satellite imagery and global positioning systems (GPS) (11). It is used to search larger geographical areas that other search methods cannot search, without placing the investigators at risk (18). Remote sensing is the optimal choice for investigators who are searching for mass graves, which are often found in areas where there are a lot of military, and rebel activity. This activity makes the area where possible clandestine mass graves are located too dangerous for investigators to do conventional search methods.

Remote sensing can be done in a multiple of ways, utilizing many different technologies. These methods include Aerial photographs, Ultraviolet (UV) photography, Infrared (IR) photography, Satellite and hyperspectral imagery, Light Detection and Ranging (LiDAR), and unmanned air vehicles (UAVs) to locate clandestine and mass graves, among other things (11). These methods are useful for locating clandestine graves because they all are non-intrusive, and can be done faster than the other search methods. Each of the remote sensing methods has their advantages and disadvantages. Some of the earlier remote sensing methods like Aerial photography can be affected by the weather, as well as tree canopy, where methods are such IR photography, UV photography and LiDAR will work regarding the weather and the geographical location of the search (11). Most of the remote sensing techniques look for a change in vegetation growth; newer, more luscious vegetation can indicate a clandestine or mass grave (11).

All of the remote sensing methods have been extensively tested and proven to be extremely successful in locating clandestine and mass graves. But a disadvantages of these methods is that the researcher's need to have an approximate knowledge of the area that needs to be searched. This knowledge can come from a number of different sources, especially for mass grave purposes, such as historical photographs and witness testimonies (18). Another disadvantage is that remote sensing can be very expensive if you do not own the tools. Most police departments do not have their own private access to planes that have this capability. However there are a few organizations such as the Royal Canadian Mounted Police (RCMP) that have full time access to remote sensing planes for searching (19). Lastly, once remote sensing has detected a clandestine or mass grave the investigators will begin excavation which can put them in danger. Due to the horrific nature of the crime, those who committed it do not want it to be found and by investigator excavating these graves can often put them in dangers way.

Remote sensing is a great searching technique; most of the methods used in remote sensing are quite successful in locating in clandestine graves. But this technique is better utilized in searching of large area in dangerous geographical locating for mass graves, rather than local clandestine graves. Although the literature states that UAVs are becoming more popular (11) and common for doing other work such as locating missing hikers. It is believed that this technique would be effective in searching local areas for clandestine graves, and as more research and studies are conducted on its effectiveness, this method will become more commonly used to locate clandestine graves.

Google Earth might be a good supplement for police forces that do not have access to remote sensing equipment to use "remote sensing" to locate clandestine graves, without the normal costs. Google Earth is a free program provided by Google that allows the user to travel the earth through a virtual globe compiled of satellite imagery, maps, terrain, and 3D buildings (20). With proper training, police investigator could use Google Earth to locate clandestine graves. There has been a study that used Google Earth in conjunction with other technologies, such as GeoEye Multispectral Imagery, to locate graves that had been looted in Peru (21). This same method, to locate looted graves could be used to locate clandestine graves, also as forensic investigators had the proper training in how to locate possible grave locating by using remote sensing.

Probing

Probing is essentially, sticking probes into the ground so that the operator can "feel" whether the soil has been disturbed, possibly indicating that there might be a grave there (11). Probing is the least expensive technologically based searching method (22). Although it is the least expensive, it might be the worst method based on the fact that it is extremely intrusive (22), which is bad for forensic investigations because it can damage or destroy the remains and crime scenes. To be able to use probing as a search method the operator must be specially trained, and must have sufficient amount of practice and experience probing (22). This is to optimistically prevent the operator from damaging the crime scene or the remains.

To use probing as a method, it requires special probes. A type of probe that can be used it called the Owsley Probe (22). Probes are generally built from a steel pole or rod that is approximately 1-2cm in diameter. The length of a probe will generally range from one to two meters long and at one end of the pole there will be a T-bar, to be used as a handle (22). The thinner the pole the more likely it will miss rocks, but you cannot have the probe too thin or it will be damaged. The length and diameter of the pole will often be dependent on the environment the operator is probing, areas with loose sandy areas and boggy areas can require a longer probe, while areas such as denser clays may require shorter probes (22). Probes will often be equipped with spring gauges or penetrometers that take measurements of the strength of soil while probing, which then can be used to grid the different strengths of the soil in the searched areas (11). When probing the investigators will document "soft spots" which are areas where the probe goes further into the soil with the same amount of pressure, and "hard spots" which are sudden sports where there is greater compaction, because this could be the result of the suspect placing branches or rocks over the remains before burying them (23).

Probing has proven to be a successful method in locating clandestine graves; it has successfully located World War II graves in Germany (11) as well as old trenches dug for pipes in Ireland (22). Although probing is successful in locating changes in soils, it is not the best method for locating clandestine graves because of how intrusive the method is.

Technological searching methods, may be some of the most efficient and successful methods for searching for clandestine graves. They are often probable and can be performed by small teams covering large areas. Despite the fact that they are so successful they still are not perfect. Many of the technological methods show more than one anomaly while surveying the search area, which can lead to investigators excavating multiple areas to exclude them. But technology is always changing and with time so will the accuracy and reliability of these methods.

Natural Methods

Not only can clandestine graves be located through canine and technological based methods, but they can be located through natural methods as well. Much like the way remote sensing looks for changes in vegetation from the sky, the same application can be attributed to ground searches as well. Such methods include Vegetation Dynamics and Forensic Taphonomy, and Soil Gas Surveying. These methods are not as used as the previous methods mention but they are starting to be utilized in searching for human remains and clandestine graves.

Taphonomy

Forensic Taphonomy is the study of the changes of an organism between the time of death and the time of discovery (24). They can use their skills to study the stages in which a human body decomposes and use this and other natural processes to locate clandestine graves (25).

Often the rate of decomposition can cause changes in the plant growth surrounding the grave. If the victim's body has some sort of drug or chemical in it, when they decompose it will be released into the surrounding soil. Such drugs can kill the surround patch of plant life, or can change the soils moisture and pH (25) killing the plants that utilize the soil.

These changes in the plant life surrounding a clandestine grave is what can be used to locate the grave. Investigators can use "environmental profiling" to help them locate graves and even connect suspects to a crime scene (26). Researchers have studied these processes to determine if they are effective at locating clandestine graves and have gotten mixed results. Some studies indicated that there is a strong difference between the growth of the vegetation before and after the grave was dug. But then other researchers have found that there was very little differences between the amount of vegetation on the grave from before and after it was dug (26). One factor that could have affected the amount of vegetation that grew on the grave site is the depth of the grave itself (26) but it is unclear as how this would affect the plant growth. Other factors that may prevent the growth of vegetation besides the depth of the graves are environmental factors such as pH levels, redox conditions, ambient temperatures, seasonality, time of burial, soil type, moisture content and local land use (27). It is clear by the literature that researchers need to do more research on this topic if they are to use it as a reliable, accurate method for locating clandestine graves. Our new understanding of decomposition and VOCs could improve this method and make it more reliable for locating clandestine graves.

Soil Gas Surveying

Forensic Taphonomy is not the only way that we can "naturally" locate clandestine graves. There have been recent advancements in using chemicals, such as methane (CH_4), to locate clandestine graves. Using chemicals have become increasingly popular; the method has become to be known as Soil Gas Surveying (28). When a "cadaver" decomposes it releases an abundance of fluids into the soil, this can create aerobic conditions, but the establishment of this aerobic condition will slow the rate of decomposition which can create the build-up of reduced gases such as methane (CH_4), and other various gases (28). When enough of these gases have built up they can diffuse into the soil and eventually be either released into the atmosphere or be subjected to oxidation (28). This process in the right condition can cause the concentration of methane to increase in the soil which then can indicate the presence of a clandestine grave (28).

To test the level of the methane gas researchers will collect both the air just above the grave and soil samples to determine the levels of methane (CH_4) gas (28). From these samples, the researchers can indicated the levels of methane, which then can be used to locate grave sites.

Based on a study that used an animal graveyard to test soil gas surveying the researchers were able to document and increase of methane (CH_4) in graves that had active decay (28). Although this study was successful in identifying the increase of methane (CH_4) in graves, this technique has not been fully tested. The study that used this method was the first study showing that using methane (CH_4) can locate graves. This method needs to be tested more before it can become a regular standard method in searching for human remains and clandestine graves. From the literature, it appears that there is no standard in collecting soil gas surveys; this can be due to the fact that this is a new technique. This method is better than a similar previously used Vapor Monitors because it is non-intrusive whereas vapor monitors are. A vapor monitor is a type of hydrocarbon detector, which is similar to the hydrocarbon detectors used by the fire department (23). They are often used in conjunction with probing but only in temperatures greater than 45°F (23). As researchers test the soil gas surveying method further, the accuracy and reliability of the technique will increase and this method may one day become a standard technique for locating human remains.

Human Searches

Canine, Geophysical and Natural methods are not the only methods that can be used to locate clandestine graves. Human powered searchers are just as useful for locating clandestine as the other methods. Visual Assessment is a method that involves walking over a designated area and scanning the ground looking for human remains or indicators of a clandestine grave, such as increases in vegetation growth, animal activity and depressions in the ground (24). Visual Assessment is not only for trained forensic investigators, but also for the public. There have been documented cases where average civilians report suspicious areas or ground disturbances that can lead to the discovery of clandestine graves (29). The civilians can often find suspicious areas, while walking their dog, in areas where there is not a lot of other civilian or police traffic. Sometime they may locate human remains, while playing fetch with their dog. Dogs have been known to accidently come back with a human bone instead of a stick. Accidental finds from civilians can be beneficial for locating clandestine graves, because civilians will often get to areas where law enforcement is less likely to get to, such as hiking paths and trails (29). There was a study conducted that looked at the number of civilians that accidently found clandestine graves (23). The researcher team viewed 788 reported homicides that involved the burial of human remains, and found that 55% of there were clandestine graves that were found by a witness reporting suspicious activity, by accident, or by the suspect giving up information (23). This study shows the how valuable civilians are to identifying the location of clandestine graves.

Civilians finding graves along trails in forests are not the only way that they can locate clandestine graves. Civilians might come into contact with clandestine graves during home improvements and renovations. There have been many documented cases of criminals hiding bodies in under concrete floors, back yards and behind walls (30). Many famous serial kills including John Wayne Gacy, Fred West, Ward Weaver and Micheal Lock all buried their victims in concrete floors (30). This is yet again another way civilians can help locate un-marked graves, and the once a suspected grave is located, other methods such as GPR can be used to confirm the graves and its exact location.

Another way humans have located clandestine graves, specifically those from mass genocide, are through complex mathematical social networks (31). The Argentine Team of Forensic Anthropology (EAAF) successfully located clandestine graves, from mass genocides that occurred in Argentina during 1976-1983 (31) using these networks. EAAF used social networking, which were made up of nodes and links to determine the location of clandestine graves and compared them against known locations of illegal detention centers (IDC) where most of these genocide killings and burials were taking place (31). Nodes represented the missing individuals, while the links represented the individual's relationships with each other, survivors and families. When each link is created it is restricted by "rules" (31). Rules are defined by functions, in which each function is based on whether there is a link between two nodes, and how much information is known about their relationship such as political attributes (31). Using these rules, nodes and functions, and mapping them against known locations of IDU the members of the EAAF were able to find clandestine graves. Complex social networking requires a great deal of mathematical background to be able to use this method to locate clandestine graves.

This method of social networking is not ideal for forensic investigators because they may not have the required background to be able to use this method to its full advantage. This method shows how civilians and survivors of mass murders can be helpful in locating the remains of the victims buried in mass clandestine graves. This method might gain more popularity if it was simplified, but since this method is location specific it would make is extremely difficult to make this it user friendly.

Conclusion

There will continue to be clandestine graves for as long as there are people committing murder. Bettering and developing methods that can locate these clandestine graves is critical for forensic investigations because without the body investigators sometime cannot make arrests for these crimes. There are currently many different methods for locating human remains and clandestine graves; they all have their advantages and disadvantages that affect their credibility and reliably when it comes to locating grave sites. But as researchers keep investigating and improving these methods, they will become better at locating clandestine graves with great ease.

This literature review looked at a number of forensic anthropological searching methods and out-lined many of their advantages and disadvantages and how successful they were in locating human remains and clandestine graves. The literature has stated "no single methodology has been successful in all conditions and geographical locations and the detection of grave..." (28). It is clear from the literature that clandestine grave search methods have become multidisciplinary. A multidisciplinary approach will help progress each method and will produce the most successful, accurate, credible and reliable searching techniques that will locate clandestine graves in all conditions and geographical locations.

Companies like NecroSearch International, combine all these different field techniques and provides the proper training, and assistance to forensic investigators around the world (32). It is a company like NecroSearch International that will help progress the current searching techniques and methods used to locate clandestine graves. Members from this company have already helped developed current methods as well as created new searching techniques. Lee Reed, a member of NecroSearch International, developed an algorithm to make searching landfills for human remains possible (32). This is an important discovery, because now forensic anthropologists and investigators can find more human remains, which can ultimately lead to more arrests and convictions.

In the future, with the help of companies like NecroSearch International, development of technology and the continual testing, that there will soon be forensic anthropological clandestine grave searching technique that will be extremely effective no matter the condition and geographical location they are used in.

References

(1) DeGreeff L, Weakley-Jones B, Furton K. Creation of training aids for human remains detection canines utilizing a non-contact, dynamic airflow volatile concentration techniques. Forensic Sci Inter 2012;217:32-8.

(2) Larson D, Vass A, Wise M. Advanced scientific methods and procedures in the forensic investigation of clandestine graves. J of Contem Crim Just 2011;27(2):149-182.

(3) Lasseter A, Jacobi K, Farley R, Hensel L. Cadaver dog and handler team capabilities in the recovery of buried human remains in the southeastern United States. J Forensic Sci 2003;48(3):1-5.

(4) Vass A, Smith R, Thompson C, Burnett M, Dulgerian N, Eckernrode B. Odor analysis of decomposing buried human remains. J Forensic Sci 2008;53(2):384-391.

(5) Vass A. Beyond the grave- understanding human decomposition. Microbio Today 2001;28:190-192.

(6) Cablk M, Sagebiel J. Field capability of dogs to locate individual human teeth. J Forensic Sci 2011;56(4):1018-1024.

(7) Migala A, Brown S. Use of human remains detection dogs for wide area search after wildfire: A new experience for Texas task force 1 and rescue resources. Wild & Enviro Med 2012(23):337-42.

(8) Fiedler S, Bernhard I, Berger J, Graw M. The effectiveness of ground-penetrating radar surveys in the location of unmarked burial sites in modern cemeteries. J Appl Geophy 2009;68(3):380-385.

(9) Novo A, Lorenzo H, Rial F, Solla M. 3D GPR in forensics: Finding a clandestine grave in a mountainous environment. Forensic Sci Int 2011;204:134-138.

(10)   Schultz J. Using ground-penetrating radar to locate clandestine graves of homicide victims: Forming forensic archaeology partnership with law enforcement. Homicide Stud 2007;11(1):15-29.

(11) Pringle J, Ruffell A, Jervis JR, Donnelly L, McKinley J, Hansen J, Morgan R, Pirrie D, Harrison M. The use of geoscience methods for terrestrial forensic searches. Earth-Sci Rev 2012;114:108-123.

(12) Pringle J, Holland C, Szkornik K, Harrison M. Establishing forensic search methodologies and geophysical surveying for the detection of clandestine graves in coastal beach environments. Forensic Sci Inter 2012;219:e29-e36.

(13) Heilig A, Eisen O, Schneebeli M. Temporal observations of a seasonal snowpack using upward-looking GPR. Hydrol Proc 2010;24:3133-3145.

(14) Solla M, Riveiro B, Alvarez M, Arias P. Experimental forensic scenes for the characterization of ground-penetrating radar wave response. Forensic Sci Inter 2012;220(1-3):50-58.

(15) Pringle J, Jervis J. Electrical resistivity survey to search for a recent clandestine burial of a homicide victim, UK. Forensic Sci Inter 2010;202:e1-e7.

(16) Jervis J, Pringle J, Tuckwell G. Time-lapse resistivity surveys over simulated clandestine graves. Forensic Science International 2009;192(1-3):1-13.

(17) Pringle J, Jervis J, Hansen J, Jones G, Cassidy N, Cassella J. Geophysical monitoring of simulated clandestine graves using electrical and ground-penetrating radar methods: 0-3 years after burial. J Forensic Sci 2012;57(6):1467-1486

(18) Kalacska M, Bell LS. Remote sensing as a tool for the detection of clandestine mass graves. Can Soc Forensic Sci J 2006;39(1):1-13.

(19) Yamashita B.Forensic Science and Identification Services: Forensic Identification. 2014,;1-102.

(20) Google. Overview of Google Earth [Internet]. Google 2014 cited March 28, 2014]. Available from: https://support-google-com.cat1.lib.trentu.ca/earth/answer/176145?hl=en English.

(21) Lasaponara R, Leucci G, Masini N, Persico R. Investigating archaeological looting using satellite images and GEORADAR: The experience in Lambayeque in North Peru. J Arch Sci 2014;42:216-230.

(22) Ruffel A. Burial location using cheap and reliable quantitative probe measurements. Forensic Sci Inter 2005;151(1-3):207-211.

(23) Gardner R. Special Scene Considerations In: Practical Crime Scene Processing and Investigation. 1st ed. CRC Press; 2005; p. 332-240.

(24) Byers, S. Introduction of Forensic Anthropology. 4th ed. Upper Saddle River, NJ: Pearson Education Inc; 2011.

(25) Carter D, Yellowlees D, Tibbett M. Moisture can be the dominant environmental parameter governing cadaver decomposition in soil. Forensic Sci Inter 2010;200:60-66.

(26) Caccianiga M, Bottacin S, Cattaneo C. Vegetation dynamics as a tool for detecting clandestine graves. J Forensic Sci 2012;57(4):983-988.

(27) Pringle J, Cassella J, Jervis J. Preliminary soilwater conductivity analysis to date clandestine burials of homicide victims. Forensic Sci Inter 2010;198:126-133.

(28) Dalva M, Kalacska M, Moore T, Costopoulos A. Detecting graves with methane. Geoderma 2012;189:18-27.

(29) Ruffell A, Donnelly C, Carver N, Murphy E, Murray E, McCambridge J. Suspect burial excavation procedure: A cautionary tale. Forensic Sci Inter 2009;183(1-3):e11-e16.

(30) Ruffell A. A search methodology for objects below and behind brick and concrete. Forensic Sci Int 2014 1-33.

(31) Caridi I, Dorso C, Gallo P, Somigliana C. A framework to approach problems of forensic anthropology using complex networks. Phys A 2011(390):1662-76.

(32) NecroSearch International. Search Methods [Internet]. 2014 [cited March 27, 2014]. Available from: http://necrosearch.org/Methods.html English.